© Copyright 2020 - All rights reserved.

TABLE OF CONTENTS

INTRODUCTION

I t has been thoroughly established that diet plays an essential role in leading and living a healthy life. Looking at the western part of the world, diet has changed over the decades. Diets that are high in cholesterol, saturated fat, sugar, salt but low in fibre are found to be one major cause of cardiovascular disease. There is a rise in the rate of obesity related diseases and most especially coronary heart in almost every part of the world. A reduction in calorie intake and food consumption without having a poor eating habit or malnutrition is believed to help promote longevity.

When a new kind of diet is introduced, almost everyone tends to be curious as to how it works and what effects it will likely have on their body, and whether or not they should give it a trial. Of recent, the most talked about diet now is the Sirtfood Diet. It was developed by two nutritionists in the United Kingdom. This diet seems to have gained prominence after the much acclaimed singer Adele revealed her new body shape and weight and people can't just stop to praise the diet that gave her such a nice figure.

Sirtfood Diet is insanely superb and contains varieties of foods in its list. It contains foods like kale, green tea, coffee, red wine, chicken, dark chocolate, extra virgin olive oil, salmon, buckwheat noodles, red onions and different kinds of condiment. The most fascinating things about this diet is the inclusion of red wine and dark chocolate. Dieters are allowed to eat dark chocolate and drink red wine on a daily basis. No restriction on the two. To most nutritionist, calories have directly linked to how people gain weight and build fat. Strict restriction on calorie intake is placed on this diet

CHAPTER ONE

THE SCIENCE BEHIND

In both humans and animals, a restriction in calorie always delays disease thereby prolonging longevity. Basically, a good diet composition enhances good health and there are hypothesis that backed the influence calorie restrictions and some dietary factors have on age-related diseases like neurodegenerative disease, cardiovascular disease, cancer, type 2 diabetes mellitus, etc. some of these dietary factors that reduces cardiovascular disease include red wine, olive oil.

Generally, calorie reduction reduces body weight and has a superb effect on plasma levels, blood pressure and cholesterol which helps in the delay or inhibition of age-related conditions. The Sirtfood Diet is very restrictive and while folding this volatile restriction, there will be a significant reduction in budget weight and body fat.

Diet plays a very essential role in both human and animal health and in the inhibition of diseases. The Institute of Human Nutrition and Food Science, Christian-Albrecht's University Of Kiel situated in Germany found that combination of both Mediterranean diet and Asian Sirtfoods diet will likely be a dietary plan in inhibiting chronic health related problems (EStruch R et al. 2013). Also, a study conducted by the Institute of Health Science, Shanghai and Green Laboratory for the science behind Aging, the Department of Biology, Massachusetts gathered that Sirtuins enable the body to burn fat to boost insulin sensitivity and energy.

Sirt Diet is premised around the intake of food which interacts with a certain class of proteins known as Sirtuins protein. The Sirtuins protein consists of seven members named SIRT1-SIRT7 respectively.

However, from a scientific point of view, little is known about this diet. The Sirtuins protein helps in regulating fat and likewise glucose metabolism based on changes in energy levels. Additionally, Sirtuins also play a vital role in how calorie restriction impact aging (Haigis MC and Guarente LP. 2006). This is likely to be because of the influence Sirtuins have on aerobic metabolism, reduction in free radicals and increment in antioxidants.

Although, SIRT1 to SIRT7 have been linked to different beneficial roles in mammals. For instance, a research shown that transgenic mice with higher percentage of SIRT6 in them have a prolonged lifespan than another type of mice, the wild mice. SIRT1, SIRT3 and SIRT4 play significant role in metabolism stimulation during food reduction or limitation. Some changes in SIRT6 reaction are also believed to stimulate the aging of some certain human skin cells. While SIRT2 is said to reduce aging in yeast.

The Sirt diet review is increasing by the day and will likely work for some people. But having a concrete scientific proof will go a long way. Howbeit, not forgetting that any scientific study on the beneficial effect that any kind of diet possesses on weight loss and other things will require a large pool of sample such as the representative of the category of population the study will focus on plus, random allocation to a control group. The outcomes would of course be on a close monitoring over a stipulated period of time, also remembering to take into account other variables that may arise. Any kind diet-based study that passes through this path will definitely be scientifically backed up and proven, but anything otherwise is not acceptable.

Tentatively, conducting this study on SIRT Diet will most likely be limited by some methods such as recollection, but would be very helpful in discovering the potency of this diet. But then, this kind of research or study does not exist for this diet.

Another thing worth mentioning is some of the claims of this diet. It claims a reduction of seven pounds in weight over a period of seven days. This is not achievable and very unrealistic. Losing seven pounds of weight won't have any effect on the body fat. When the body experiences energy deprivation, it utilizes either glycogen or its stored emergency energy and this is in addition to muscle loss and fat burning.

For glycogen, each of its molecules needs about 3-4 water molecules for it to be stored. When the body makes use of this glycogen, the water is gotten rid of too and this is termed **water weight.**

Hence, during the first week of rigorous calorie restriction, just a few of the weight loss comes directly from fat while the remaining weight loss is from muscle, water and glycogen. However, the moment there's an increase in your calorie intake, your body regains its glycogen back and then, your weight returns.

Sadly enough, this form of calorie restriction can make your body reduce its metabolic rate which will eventually make you need fewer calories on a daily basis for energy. There's every possibility that this diet will help you to lose weight during the first few weeks, but the weight will definitely come right back as soon as you end the diet.

For the inhibition of health related conditions, following the diet on a course of three weeks is never going to make any positive impact compared to when it's a long term procedure. But combining your daily diet with Sirtfoods over a long period of time will be a good idea.

Generally, applying scientific method to nutritional study is always difficult. Research design often time is very hard and challenging because conducting placebo control trail with just any level of ecological validity is not possible and the health outcomes researchers always look forward to occurs over a long of years. In a nutshell, SIRT Diet is not very certain to offer any health benefits to people suffering from diabetes, hiding in the shadow of obesity. As indicated by some people, special diet is not effective and dieting as a whole is not a general public solution for communities where more than half of its adults population is suffering from obesity.

CHAPTER TWO

THE SKINNY GENE

What is the Skinny Gene?

For the majority of us who find our body shape and size so unattractive and unappealing. We are disturbed about how we can control, contour and change our body shape. Have we ever considered the possibility that what if the ability to change this does not lie in our hands?

One way or the way, we must have come across people that no matter how much the quantity of food they eat, they never seem to add up weight. Many studies and research have been conducted as to how some people don't ever seem to gain an iota of pounds irrespective of the way they eat, while others gain weight at an alarming rate. Well, the answer lies in our genes.

The perfect genes are rare to come by. When talking about weight gain and obesity or even when conducting a research or study on the two, genetics must be properly considered as they play essential role in both obesity and weight gain. Some people are blessed with the skinny gene and they are able to turn it on while others are not so lucky. Even if you fall into the category of those who are unlucky, there are things you can do to turn on and turn off the gene as you want. Funny right? The secret is what is termed **gene interaction**.

Gene interaction is the process of improving how your gene interacts with your environment.

Sirtuins otherwise known as the skinny gene is very active in changing how cells function. Sirtuins are potent in burning fat. They are a special kind of gene reason being that they can turn our cells into a survival mode. This is done through a process called autophagy. This process also gets rid of cellular waste and unwanted particles that store up over time which end up causing inflammaging (Riveros-McKay et al. 2019). The end result of this restoration process is alarming – our body cells become younger looking, healthy and better while inflammation becomes a thing of the past. Activating this gene is what brings about weight loss and prevention of health related issues in people.

Sirtuin Activating Compounds

There are some foods that can activate Sirtuins in the body. However, the amount needed to activate sirtuin in Human is not yet known. These activators tend to elevate insulin sensitivity and reduces blood sugar levels to a greater extent. The sirtuin activators are said to be the following natural molecules.

I.   Polyphenols- Present in turmeric, curcumin. Moderate amount is needed to have a beneficial effect in the body. Consuming a high amount of it can be dangerous.

II.   Resveratrol- present in blueberries, red grade, raspberries and peanuts. Helps in combating inflammation and improving heart health.

III. Quecertin- Present in apples, kale, capers, berries, onion, citrus fruits and helps in combating inflammation.

IV.   Piceatannol- Popularly used as herbal medicine in Asian countries. It's present in red wine, white etc.

V.   Oligonol- Rich in anti-inflammatory properties and often present in lychees.

VI.   Fisetin- improves long term memory and present in strawberries.

VII.   Omega-3- present in flaxseeds, fish like salmon, catfish, tilapia etc.

VIII.   Melatonin.

Consuming any foods sources of the above mentioned compounds can activate sirtuin proteins in your body.

Paradoxically, there are other ways that the skinny gene can be turned on which is through fasting and exercise (Radak et al 2013). This can be a very difficult thing to do for most people considering their busy schedule which in most cases never leave time for exercise and fasting. The aftermath of fasting is nothing but a feeling of hunger and anger which can cause stagnation in metabolism. Talking about physical exercise, the amount required for weight loss depends on the amount of strength and effort that's been put into it.

Scientific Study on Skinny Gene

Twin studies have indicated that weight variation is highly caused by genetics. Nowadays, lots of research have focused on people that are obese. A study was conducted by Professor Farooqi and his team to examine the real reason behind why some people remain thin and others do not. The study comprises 14,000 participants out of which there were 1,622 thin men and women. 1,985 obese people and over 10,000 people with normal weight. The DNA of these people were compared. So, why studying the genes for this?

The truth is, our DNA consists of proteins that are responsible for some particular functions in our body system. Any kind of change in this gene called genetic variant, can form another kind of protein and thus, altering the function of the protein within the body. If it's a protein that involves in metabolism, there will be changes in the way our body processes and digests food and even stores them.

Going further, the team was able to identify some genetic variants that have the ability to increase people's risk of being obese. They were also able to find a novel genetic region that explains why some people are thin (Riveros-McKay et al. 2019). The impact these genetic variants have on individual's weight were created in a risk score. It was discovered that thin individuals have a significantly low genetic risk score. The result proved that vibrant thin individuals are thin because they possess a lower genes burden that decreases a person's chance of being obese or overweight and not because they were created perfectly.

The belief of people for the past few years is that genetic is a causal factor of most diseases like cancer, obesity and so on. Scientifically, genetics play just 10 percent role in the risk of these diseases while the remaining 90 percent is dependent on environmental factors. Surprised right? The way we sleep, eat, walk, behave, drink, reason and talk are all your environmental factors that you have control over.

In older adults, weight gain is a major determinant of how quickly they are aging. The fact that your body functions with the 90/10 rule makes it even easier for you to make good use of the genes at your disposal. There are some genes called **famine.** These are genes that work to assist you extract as much energy as they can from the food you consume. Thereby, giving you the ability to store fat and live through famine.

You could have called this a brilliant idea some years back unlike now that these same genes can add to your weight. Although, 75 genes play a major role in becoming obese, there are major ones that can increase your risk of obesity and weight gain. There are also ways in which you can control these genes and activate them as you wish. Not minding the fact that these genes are a part of you, there are ways you can control them, you have the power to decide how they interact and relate within your body.

Genes Associated With Weight Gain

There are certain genes that are associated with weight again which are responsible for how people gain weight unnecessarily mainly because of their eating habit. Some of these genes include:

Fat Mass and Obesity (FTO GENE)

This is the gene that has the strongest link with your body mass index. It's your greatest risk of diabetes and obesity. There's a variant that switches on the gene and if this variant is present in your body, you will not be able to control the hormone of satiety called leptin. Thus, making you to eat unnecessarily. The FTO gene acts like a fat sensor and people with this kind of gene tend to eat excessively most especially fatty foods, particularly in childhood. People who share an abnormal gene from the two parents weigh more and are at the greater risk of becoming obese. While people with normal gene have a lower risk of obesity.

The FTO gene can be switch on with adequate and proper physical exercise. Making sure you sleep between 7 to 8 hours at night, consuming low carbohydrates food and increasing your higher fibre intake. With proper dietary and good lifestyle, your risk of obesity can be reduced.

Melancortin 4 Receptor

People born with this gene will consume more of snacks even if they are not hungry. They spend much of their time eating between meals, snacking on cake, chips and so on. This gene increases the urge for fat.

If you have an increasing urge for snack, simply learn to eat three times daily. Eat at intervals of four to six hours between each meal, with no snacking in between. Don't rush when eating. Set a boundary for your food consumption so you can easily combat the food addiction.

Adrenergic beta-2 Surface Receptor

This is a different kind of famine and it's associated with the distribution of fat. When this gene is turn on, the gene can hinder your body fat from breaking down, resulting in slower metabolic rate thus, making you store fat. This famine gene can increase your risk of obesity three times over. It can also increase the risk of type 2 diabetes. Also, people with this kind of gene find it really difficult to lose weight.

How do you deal with this gene? It's simple. Exercise is one of the possible solutions. Accept the fact that losing weight will be difficult for you so, don't feel bad when you see another person losing weight better and faster than you. Be disciplined in your eating habit. Eat the right kind of food with the right amount of nutrients. This is a slow and steady mission so you mustn't rush it.

What are the Roles Of Gut Bacteria in Genes?

According to trails conducted on gut bacteria, result have shown that the existence of some bacteria are associated with different kind of body weight in people and how this works is not well understood yet. What is known is that these bacteria can produce chemicals that can change people's genes.

Gut bacteria can be influenced right from birth and babies born with Caesarean are found to have a different kind of balance from those born naturally. There are some steps you can take to enhance your gut bacteria's health whilst, stimulating your weight.

The Importance Of Diet

A lot of researchers have developed a keen interest in how genes work and react, the genes we have and the ones we are lacking in. The fact still remains that we are stuck with our individual genetic makeup, take it or leave it. One thing we should know is that these genes can be influenced in some ways. How?

Nutrition could turn on and turn off genes

Firstly, the kind of environment will find ourselves and the kind of food we eat can have a significant effect on our genes. The skinny gene is believe to be present in everybody which means we just have to find it and turn it on.

It's not all about the genetic factor

It's very possible that some people are being exposed to certain things due to their genetic makeup in the aspect of body weight and many other factors. Genes can actually be overcome if it's the main cause of your body weight. With the right diet and exercise, genes can be overcome. When this is done in the proper way and manner, it's very possible you lose all this weight troubling you.

Put no blames on the genes for the increase in obesity

Why blame your genetic makeup for your being obese? As stated above that genes play just 10 percent role in the risk of obesity while the remaining 90 percent is caused by environmental factors. Why not analyze these factors and make adjustments where needed, rather than blaming your genes for your overweight problem?

Sirtfood Diet

CHAPTER THREE

BURNING FAT

If it appears to you that the excess calories intake you consume stores in your belly or thighs, you are really not assuming wrongly. You are very right about this. The belly and thighs are the most targeted places for fat storage and this is mostly due to some factors such as age, genes, lifestyle, body type, hormones and also how our bodies process, store and get rid of fat, and so on.

Sometimes, your body stores calories as fat just to keep you hale and healthy. The issue most people usually face about this is how to get rid of the excess fat.

By and large, millions of people have adopted uncountable ways to get rid of the extra fat in their body by practicing one or two of the burning gimmicks they've heard of or read on the internet that includes the use of supplement, consumption of certain foods, spot reduction and many more.

Low amount of body fat is as dangerous as having a high amount of it. The body needs a specific amount of fat so it can function maximally as it should. For women, the ideal percentage of body fat is about 10 to 13 percent, while for men, it's about 2 to 5 percent. Having below this level can lead to unfavourable conditions like, for instance, nervous system issue, vitamin deficiencies, diabetes, risk of heart disease, low immunity, infertility etc.

In addition, lack of body fat tends to breakdown and weaken the muscles which will automatically make you feel weak and tired.

Essentials of Fat Burning

If you are working on losing weight, you are expected that knowing how your body consumes calories for energy and fuel can make a significant difference in how deal with your weight loss goal. Energy is gotten from three major classes of foods; protein, carbohydrates and fat respectively. The one that your body gets energy from depends solely on the kind of activity you engage in.

Often time, majority of people prefers to use fat for their body fuel or energy, this is good. You become aware that the more fat you expend as energy or fuel, the lesser the fat you will have stored up in your body. However, expending these fat doesn't necessarily mean you are losing that body fat. To truly have the in-depth understanding of how to burn fat, you need to first of all know where your body takes its energy from. That is, you need to figure out the source of your energy.

Basically, both carbs and fat are the primary sources of the body's fuel. With a little amount of protein used during exercise or physical activity. Protein is also mostly used to repair worn out tissues and replenish muscles after exercise. Thus, the proportion of these so called fuels will change based on the kind of exercise you are doing.

During higher intensity activities, like briskly running, sport like football, fast cycling and so on, the body uses more of carbs for fuel compared to fat. You may wonder why? This is simply because the metabolic pathways that are responsible to breakdown carbohydrates for energy are highly efficient than the pathways responsible for fat breakdown. While for a light to moderate intensity physical activities, fat is used as fuel in the body than carbohydrates.

In weight loss, what you should be concerned about is how to burn more calories and not how to use more fat for energy. The higher the intensity of your exercise, the higher the calories you tend to burn. In essence, the fact that you are expending more fat as fuel doesn't necessarily mean you are burning more calories.

Fat Burning Zone Theory

The fat burning zone theory started based on the believe that light intensity activities consume more fat than carbs for energy. And this birthed the idea that when you exercise at a particular heart rate zone out of the maximum heart rate zone, like 55 to 65 percent out of 100 percent will enable your body to burn a higher percentage of fat.

This is a very misleading notion. We so much believe in this theory that we have programmed our exercise around it. Exercising at low or moderate intensities is not such a bad idea. It won't burn more fat except you are burning more calories than you consume. In order to burn more calories, you will need to workout at higher intensities.

Burning Fat and Cardio

Cardio is believed to be very hard. Some people even believed that cardio is all about high intensity activity. Variety they say is the spice of life. You can include some variety which can help you to regulate your various energy systems and this will enable you to derive pleasure in your workouts. This way, you can design cardio program that comprises varieties of activities at various intensities.

Pros of High Intensity Activities

- It increases metabolic rate.
- It's effective for weight loss.
- It can reduce blood sugar level.
- Enhances energy consumption.
- It supports muscle building.
- Reduces heart rate and blood pressure.
- Burns calories faster.

Cons of High Intensity Activities

As effective as high-intensity activities are in burning fat, it is not without its own risk. They include:

- Overuse injuries
- Developing hatred for exercise
- Burnout
- Overtraining
- Inconsistent exercise

Pros of Moderate Intensity Activities

- It promotes better health by reducing the risk of diabetes, cancer, heart disease, stroke and high blood pressure.
- It has more varieties of activities to choose from.

- Allows you to workout at a comfortable pace.

- It helps to build up strength and endurance.

- Improve sleep quality.

- It boosts mood.

- Improve memory.

Pros of Low Intensity Activities

- Not challenging and taxing.

- Very comfortable.

- Improves your body's ability to use fat for fuel during exercise.

- Enhances our cardio health.

- Easier to endure.

- Stimulates faster recovery.

Cons of Low Intensity Activities

- You won't be able to build strong bones and muscles.

- Overuse injuries.

- It doesn't burn fat and calorie fast enough. Thus, it's time taken.

- Boredom.

Lift Weight to Shed Weight

Lifting weight with other resistance exercise can help you to shed body fat. This will even be more effective if you are on a diet. Many people are used to engaging in cardio exercise to burn fat, making strength training important in any weight loss program. Lifting weight helps to get rid of cancer, belly fat, heart disease and stress. It also makes you look sexy in a bikini. Below are the reasons you should embrace lifting weight to burn excess body fat.

- It makes your clothes to fit better on you.
- It increases the amount of calories you burn.
- It will improve your diet.
- It will improve your heart health.
- It will improve your mood and makes you become happier.
- You will achieve your desired body shape faster.
- You will lose more fat.
- You will have stronger bones.
- You'll become more productive and smarter.
- Gives you the ability to deal with stressful situations better.
- It will increase your lifespan.

How Do You Burn Fat Without Losing Muscles?

With the presence of muscle mass, it will be easier and faster to burn fat. Some studies have proven that fast weight loss brings about more muscle loss compared to a steady weight loss. Don't get overwhelmed counting calories or restricting it. Instead, focus your attention on maintaining your lovely muscles.

Don't get preoccupied with the scale. This is because muscles weigh higher than fat. What you read on the scale might discourage and mislead you. It's better to use a tape measure to track your body measurement and always jot it down in a notebook.

Good Fat, Bad Fat

Fats are not created the same. Some fats are good and some are bad, really bad such as the trans fats. Fat spends longer time to digest whilst, your stomach remains full for a longer time. With fat, hunger is suppressed just like protein. It digests at a slow pace thus, keeping you full for some time. Do away with the bad fats and consume the good fat. Even the good fats should be consumed moderately because they are super rich in calories. Examples of healthy fatty foods include:

1. Nuts
2. Olive oil
3. Seeds
4. Avocado
5. Coconut oil

Say No To Refined Carbs

High consumption of refined carbs is not healthy for the body and doesn't help in burning fat instead, it builds up fat. Refined carbs have passed through a refining process whereby all its vital nutrients have been stripped off. Too much of refined carbs can result into fat gain, most especially the visceral fat. When you reduce the amount of refined carbs you consume, you are automatically helping yourself to reduce the amount of fat storage in your body.

Refined carbs have high glycemic index. They can also elevate blood sugar level which will make you hungry and angry at the same time. Most fancy and classy foods we always salivate for are full of refined carbs such as cereals, pastries and pastas.

There are alternatives to refined carbs. You can switch to whole grains. They are healthy and delicious. Examples are:

1. Whole wheat
2. Barley
3. Whole grain
4. Oats
5. Quinoa

Consume more of Fibre

Fibre digests slowly in the digestive system, making you feel full for a long period of time. Eating foods high in fibre will improve your general wellbeing and at the same time, gives you a moderate body weight.

According to a study, consuming foods rich in fibre is said to help participants lose over 4.6 pounds over a period of four months. High fibre foods include the following:

1. Vegetables
2. Fruits
3. Nuts and seeds
4. Whole grains

Don't Forget Coffee

Coffee is superb and very good for the body. It contains a high amount of caffeine which aids fat burning and weight loss. It also helps in regulating the nervous system, increases metabolism rate, dissolves fat. Coffee can increase your energy level which is exactly what you need to get through with your busy schedule.

No More Carbonated Drinks and Alcohol

Sugary drinks and alcohol are close ally to body fat. They both contain a high percentage of calories. They also increase visceral fat (belly fat). Alternatively, you can switch to green tea, a glass of water, lemon water, coffee etc. They are well loaded with antioxidants which are good for the immune system and are very effective in burning body fat.

In conclusion, other ways to burn fat include the intake of iron, which you can either get from supplement or foods such as seafood, dried fruits, meat, green leafy vegetables and fortified grains. Another method is getting enough sleep. A good quality sleep of about seven hours is enough to burn those fats and lose those weight. Irrespective of your reason to want to burn fat and lose weight, just do it the right way as explained above. Doing it the wrong way can affect you overall wellbeing.

CHAPTER FOUR

THE IMPORTANCE OF EXERCISE

E xercise is very important for a healthy living, but many of us are oblivion to what we can gain from exercising. Our bodies have evolved over time and are designed to be continuously active.

Just as a vehicle is designed to move fast, humans are also designed to act and move. If a vehicle is left for long without using it on a regular basis, it tends to develop engine faults and wear out quickly.

Over time, humans too develop health issues if they remain inactive for a period of time. Sitting down for a long time at a desk or watching the tv all day reduced the amount of exercise you engage in.

What is an Exercise?

An exercise can be defined as any kind of movement that requires physical activity which works your muscles and allows your body to burn fat. There are several physical activities that make one become active such as dancing, swimming, walking, running, jogging and so on. Exercise has many benefits, be it mentally or physically, that can make you live a prolonged life.

Physical exercises promote a healthy living and prevent the occurrence of health related conditions such as a reduction in the risk of cardiovascular disease, diabetes, cancer and so on. Both exercise and physical activity have both long-term and instant impact on the general well-being. Essentially, regular exercise can enhance your quality of life. A 20 to 30 minutes exercise on a daily basis will enable you to enjoy a quality life and enjoy all the benefits associated with regular exercise.

Benefits of Regular Exercise

1. It promotes happiness

Exercise has been proven to boost mood and reduce anxiety, stress and the feeling of depression. It produces certain changes in the parts of the brain that stimulate stress and anxiety. It likewise has the ability to maximize brain sensitivity for serotonin and norepinephrine hormones that provide relief for depression.

Also, physical exercise can promote the production of endorphins which promote positive feelings and reduces the feeling of pain. Over the years, exercise has proven to be effective in reducing anxiety symptoms in people. It enables them to be mentally aware of their mental state and are able to get distracted from their fears.

Whether your physical activity is intense or not doesn't really matter, the fact still remains that your mood has a lot to benefit if you engage in exercise irrespective of its intensity.

According to a study conducted on 24 women who were suffering from depression, it was found that physical activity of any kind of intensity reduced the feelings of depression to a greater extent.

Exercise has such a significant effect on mood to the extent that whether you choose to engage in physical exercise or not will tell over a period of time. A study was conducted on 26 men and women who usually engage in physical activity on a daily basis. They were told to either keep up with the exercise or stop for a period of two weeks. The group that stopped exercising recorded an increase in negative mood.

The bottom line is, practicing regular exercise will boost your mood and minimize feelings of depression, stress and anxiety.

2.   Effective in weight loss

A lot of studies and research have shown that lack of physical activity or exercise is a causal factor in obesity and excess weight.
There exist a relationship between exercise and energy usage.

The body expend energy in three distinct ways: diversion of food, physical activity and maintenance of body functions such as breathing, thinking, heartbeat and so on.
It's evident that through dieting, calorie restriction or reduction will definitely reduce your metabolic rate, which will slow down weight reduction.

Contrarily, regular physical activity has proven to boost metabolic rate, which can get rid of more calories and boost weight reduction. To prevent weight gain and maintain the weight loss, aerobic exercise coupled with resistance training is essential in promoting fat loss and maintaining muscle mass.

Needless to say, exercise is vital in fast metabolism and in getting rid of calories on a regular basis. It's also crucial in the maintenance of both weight loss and muscle mass.

3. Reduces the Risk of Chronic Health Related Conditions

The major cause of most health issues is the lack of physical exercise. Practicing exercise increases insulin sensitivity, body functions and composition, cardiovascular health and fitness and at the same time, reduces blood pressure etc.

Lack of physical activity can increase the risk of type 2 diabetes due to the fact that lack of regular exercise can boost belly fat which happens to be a risk factor for diabetes, untimely death and heart problem.

Thus, it's advisable to engage in a regular physical exercise so as to combat the risk of developing any of these health issues.

4. It has a Positive Effect on Pain

Chronic pain tends to weaken even the strongest man, with exercise this can be reduced. In the past, the best possible way to treat chronic pain and all kinds of pain was to simply rest and avoid strenuous activity and if possible, avoid any kind of activity whatsoever, whether strenuous or not.

But now, reverse is the case as some studies have shown that exercise helps in combating chronic pain. Many studies have been able to indicate the effect exercise has in reducing chronic pain in people suffering from various kinds of health related issues such as shoulder disorder, low back pain, and so on. Most importantly, physical exercise is said to boost pain tolerance and perception in people.

5. **Helps in the Prevention of Some Cancers**

Keeping your body physically fit can reduce the risk of some cancers like breast cancer, lung cancer, colon cancer and most likely endometrial cancer too. Some studies conducted by the Seattle Cancer Research Centre have shown that most cancer deaths are caused by excess weight gain and sedentary.

6. **Promote brain health and memory**

Exercise is good for the brain and memory. It also boosts the heart rate which in turns increases the flow of blood and oxygen to the brain. Additionally, it regulates the production and supply of hormones that boost the growth and development brain cells.

In older adults, regular physical activity is a must for them. This is simply because of aging which oftentimes occurs with inflammation and oxidative stress. Engaging in exercise will enhance certain changes in the brain function and structure.

Also, regular exercise has proven to be essential for memory and learning. It increases the size of hippocampus in the human brain. Hippocampus is a component part of the brain that's responsible for learning and memory. Thus, helping to promote mental function in older people.

7. **Stimulates the Immune System**

Regular exercise enables the body to pump oxygen and essential nutrients in the body and this is needed to fuel the body cells and in getting rid of bacteria and viruses that attack the body.

8. **Promote better relaxation and sleep**

When you exercise regularly, you tend to experience a soothing and positive change in the manner at which you sleep and relax. When you sleep after having gone through a vigorous exercise, the energy you expend is replenished back. Also, when you exercise, your body temperature increases and this helps to ensure you have a good quality sleep as it decreases when you sleep.

Numerous studies have been conducted to ascertain the significant impact that exercise has on quality sleep and surprisingly, they all have the same conclusions.

A certain study showed that 120 minutes of average to vigorous physical activity on a weekly basis can enhance sleep quality by 65 percent.

Another study conducted on 17 people suffering from insomnia found that up to 16 weeks of physical exercise helped these people to sleep better unlike the control group. It also boosts their energy to partake in their daily activities during the day.

In older people suffering from sleep disorder, engaging in physical activity will improve their sleep quality and allow them to sleep longer and better.

Depending on your choice, it's either you engage in only aerobic exercise or you combine it with resistance training, there will still be an improvement in your sleep quality.

9. **It boost sex life**

Exercise promotes sex drive and libido. Regular exercise makes cardiovascular system to become stronger, increases blood flow and circulation, promotes flexibility and tone muscles, which are essential for sex life.
Some group of women in their forties state that they experienced multiple orgasms better when they engaged in aerobic exercise such as running, jogging and others.

In a group of about 200 physical fit men, the ones that engaged more in regular exercise on a weekly basis claimed they have higher sex drive and increased libido and that they were able to perform better sexually.

Another study comprising of 45 men who were asked to engage in about ten minutes walk around their houses saw a significant reduction in erectile dysfunction.

Summarily, exercise is powerful in improving sex drive in both men and women of all ages. And is very effective in reducing erectile dysfunction.

10. **Promote better skin health**

Some skins are very sensitive while others are normal. Oxidative stress can have major negative effect on the body. People experience oxidative stress when their body's antioxidants is ineffective in repairing damages done by free radicals cause by the body cells. This can result into a major damage in the internal structure of the skin and thereby, worsening the skin.

Engaging in a strenuous exercise can lead to oxidative stress. In this case, a moderate exercise is advised. Moderate to mild exercise can boost the formation of natural antioxidants which are vital in protecting the body cells. Exercise also has anti-aging effect when done moderately.

11. **Boost Energy Levels**

Regular physical exercise promotes energy levels. It's an energy booster for both the healthy ones and those suffering from one sickness or the other.

A particular study comprising of 38 men who complained about frequent fatigue indicated that six weeks of non-stop physical activity decreased fatigue.

For people suffering from chronic fatigue syndrome and other kinds of chronic sickness can experience energy level increase if they engage in a regular exercise.

12. **Good for Strong Bones and Muscles**

Exercise is an important activity when looking into building strong bones and muscles. With the consumption of the right amount of protein and vigorous exercise like weight lifting will boost muscle building. When you exercise, the hormone that allows your muscles to absorb amino acids is released into your body. Thus, allowing the muscles to grow whilst, inhibiting their breakdown.

The more people grow and age, the faster they lose muscle function and mass which makes them prone to disabilities and injuries. Engaging in regular exercise is effective in combating muscle loss as you become older.

How Much Exercise Do You Really Need?

The American College Of Sports Medicine in their guidelines stated that for people between the ages of 19 to 64 to stay fit and healthy, they should make sure they are active every day. The following recommendations were provided:

a. Cardiorespiratory exercise , otherwise known as cardio is any kind of physical activity that enhances the heartbeat and breathing rate. Example we have walking, jogging, cycling, running, dancing, swimming, sports like football, basketball, volleyball and so on.

b. Resistance exercise is involved with working the muscle groups and strength building. Adults are advised to train each of the muscle group two to three times in a week with the use of various kinds of exercise and gears.

Mild and moderate intensity resistance training is ideal for older people or people that are new to exercise. It's also stated that adults should test for about 48 hours between this kind of training.

Differences Between Moderate and Vigorous Intensity

The differences between moderate and vigorous intensity are often done using heart rate, metabolic rate and perceived exertion.

Generally, moderate intensity exercise should actually increase the heart rate, followed by faster breathing, warm and sweaty. They include: dancing, swimming, brisk walking, volleyball, double tennis, slow cycling etc.

Vigorous intensity exercise on the other hand is accompanied by a very increased heart rate, hard breathing, hot temperature and excessively sweaty. They include: running, martial arts, skipping, faster cycling, power walking, aerobics, football, basketball, etc.

Based on America Physical Activity Guidelines, with moderate intensity exercise, you will only be able to talk and not sing. While the vigorous intensity exercise makes you unable to say a few words without stopping to catch a breath.

In conclusion, exercise has lots of healthy benefits that can promote almost every area of your life, if not all, both internal and external. Any activity that increases your heart rate, makes you breath faster, makes you sweat profusely and that you feel happy to do over and over again is considered great for you in every aspect.

CHAPTER FIVE

SIRTFOODS

What are Sirtfoods?

According to the nutritionist Rob Hobson Sirtfoods mean foods high in Sirtuins activators. Sirtuins are a group of proteins that help to protect the body cells from damaging, getting inflammed and dying through sickness and disease. Scientific research has also proven that they also work to enhance the body muscle, regulate metabolism rate and also burn fat.

Are Sirtfoods The Revolutionary Superfoods?

It's not a mere say that Sirtfoods are lovely and good for everyone. They are high in nutrients and packed with healthy compounds and properties.

Few studies have been able to recommend that Sirtfoods have lots of healthy benefits. For instance, consuming a right amount of dark chocolate rich in cocoa content have the tendency to minimize the risk of heart disease and help get rid of inflammation.

Also, green tea is very potent in combating the risk of stroke and even all types of diabetes and likewise effective in lowering blood pressure.

Additionally, turmeric on the other hand is high in anti-inflammatory properties and well packed with high beneficiary effects on the body and has the ability to guide the body against all forms of health related conditions. Most Sirtfoods have proven to have major beneficiary effects in humans.

There seems to be no concrete evidence on the beneficiary effects of increased level of sirtuin proteins in humans. But certain research in cell lines and other animals has proven to be beneficial. For instance, an increase in the level of a certain Sirtuins protein level leads to prolonged lifespan in worms, yeast and mice.

And in the process of calorie restriction, sirtuin proteins notify the body to burn more fat in order to gain more energy and enhance insulin sensitivity. A certain study in mice stated that an increase in Sirtuins levels result into fat loss.

Other evidence also suggests that Sirtuins plays a vital role in minimizing inflammation, preventing the growth and development of tumors and reducing the growth and development of heart related disease and Alzheimer's.

Studies in humans and mice cell lines have indicated positive outcomes, but there are no human studies yet to state the impact that increased Sirtuins levels have in humans. Thus, there is no concrete evidence to ascertain that increment in Sirtuins protein levels in humans will bring about a prolonged lifespan or reduce the risk of cancer.

There's an ongoing research on the development of compounds that will be potent at increasing Sirtuins protein levels in the human body. Due to this, studies are ongoing to know the impacts of Sirtuins in the human body.

Health Benefits of SIRTFOOD

Many evidence have been gathered which proved that Sirtuins activators are very likely to have some health benefits such as suppressing hunger, improve memory, better control of blood sugar, repairing of damages caused by free radicals, reduction in the risk cancer, diabetes and heart disease and enhancing of muscle building, to name a few.

Based on the words of an expert in nutrition and epidemiology Professor Frank Hu, Harvard University, he mentioned that there are enough evidence that proved consuming food and drink high in Sirtuins activators have beneficial effects on chronic health issues. Sirtfood Diet is exceptionally good for anti-aging.

However, Sirtuins activators are present in most planets but some fruits and vegetables have a higher amount of the protein present in them and are only considered as sources of Sirtfood. Example; kale, Indian turmeric, green tea, onions cocoa powder and parsley.

One major benefit of eating meals high in Sirtuins is mainly because they are very flexible than any other meals. It's either you add them to other meals or you eat them as a whole.

Sirtfoods encourages fat burning and muscle growth. In the weight loss regime of some diet, its usually occurs that you burn fat and lose muscle, but with Sirtfood, it's not so. You burn fat and gain more muscle. It also helps to maintain and repair muscle.

Another health benefit of eating Sirtfood is adequate supply of fibre and polyphenols which is good for the heart.

CHAPTER SIX

THE SIRTFOOD DIET

Sirtfood Diet was developed in the United Kingdom by two nutritionists who were working at a private gym. They marketed the diet as a **"revolutionary new diet"** and health strategy that works by switching on the **"skinny gene"** in the human body system.

The Sirtfood diet is the latest way to burn extreme body fat and lose weight dramatically without having to experience malnutrition or starve oneself. Activating the skinny gene is achieved through exercising and fasting. There are some categories of foods that have chemicals known as polyphenols that when consumed, they put little stress on the body cells. Thus, producing genes that imitate the consequences of both fasting and exercise. Certain foods have high polyphenols present in them such as dark chocolate (cocoa), coffee, red wine, kale and so on. When these kinds of foods are taken, they tend to release Sirtuins reactions that influence aging, mood and metabolism. Any diet high in Sirtfoods triggers weight loss without necessarily having to expend muscles, while at the same time maintaining a healthy lifestyle and health.

This particular diet focuses on calorie restriction which is in phases. This calorie restriction is believed to increase the production of Sirtuins in the body.

Is Sirtfood Diet Good For You?

Every food on the diet plan is very healthy for you. You stand to get the right amount of nutrients, vitamins, minerals and which will likely become high when following this diet. This diet is very restrictive on some kinds of foods and calories and this may make it a bit difficult for some people to follow and get accustomed to.

Is It Effective?

The developers of the diet are so positive about the wonders this diet performs in weight loss, in burning fat, in activating the body skinny gene and in the inhibition of health related conditions. The only concern is there's little proof to back these..

Conversely, there is no convincing proof to ascertain the beneficiary effects of the diet on weight loss than any other kind of calorie restricted food or diet. Nonetheless, many of the foods in this diet are rich in nutrients, minerals and vitamins but no human studies to ascertain whether consuming a diet high in Sirtfoods has any reasonable healthy benefits.

Contrarily to this, the Sirtfood Diet book states the results derived from a pilot study the authors conducted which involved 39 participants from their gym. The result of this study was not published in any other book or website except their book.

For the first week, the participants were put on strict daily diet and exercise. By the end of the first week, the participants have recorded an average of 7 pounds weight loss. Achieving this result is not surprising at all, reason being that restricting your calorie consumption to 1,000 calories coupled with exercise will result into weight loss.

Nonetheless, this kind of weight loss is not genuine and long lasting. There was no evidence to determine if there was any follow up to know whether the participants gained back the weight, which is most likely to be the case. The key to this kind of diet is continuity. You have to keep following this diet until you have achieved your desired weight goal and then keep maintaining it over and over again. In the absence of this, the moment you make a sudden swerve from this diet, you are very much likely to gain those weight back.

When the body experiences energy deprivation, it utilizes either glycogen or its stored emergency energy and this is in addition to muscle loss and fat burning.

In a nutshell, Sirtfood Diet is likely to help you lose weight virtually because it's low in calories. But be prepared to gain the weight back once the diet is over. This is because the diet is very short to have a long term effect on your body.

Sirtfood Diet Essentials

The diet consists of twenty highly rated foods, which you can combine with your everyday meal.

I. **Buckwheat:** This is available in form of noodles and fruit seed. It's in every way different from wheat. So when getting yours, it should be 100 percent buckwheat.

II. **Celery:** Very nutritious especially the hearts and the leaves. Always blend hem together.

III. **Extra virgin olive oil:** This is a very top ingredient in SIRTFOOD DIET. It has a peppery taste and it's highly sirtifying.

IV.   **Bird's eye chilli:** Also known as Thai's chilli. They are more hot than regular chilis and has more nutrients.

V.   **Capers:** Good for salad.

VI.   **Green tea or matcha:** Very soothing when combined with a slice of lemon.

VII. **Cocoa:** Helps in the control of blood sugar, cholesterol and blood pressure.

VIII. **Kale:** It's a very high SIRTUINS activator. Rich in quercetin and kaempferol.

IX.   **Parsley:** Sprinkle it on your meals, juice or smoothie. It's far more than just a mere garnish.

X.   Lovage

XI.   Red onion

XII. Strawberries

XIII. Chicory

XIV. Turmeric

XV.   Soy

XVI. Red wine

XVII. Walnuts

XVIII. Soy

XIX. Medjool dates

XX.   Rocket

Does Sirtfood Diet Have Any Side Effects?

First and foremost, the diet has no room for substitutions. Sirtfood Diet is very limiting and restrictive. It counts calories and focuses on a certain food category. Even though the SIRTFOOD recommended meals may look yummy and tasty, the diet is likely to be deficient in major nutrients like iron, zinc and calcium. They are not the kind of meal you will most likely find on the "list of healthy food" says an anonymous nutritionist. Eating a little bar of chocolate and having a glass of red wine is no bad thing and won't affect the body in any way. However, it shouldn't be an everyday thing. Eating varieties of fruits and vegetables is better and not just the ones recommended on the list.

In addition, the weight loss can only be maintained only if the calorie restriction is also maintained otherwise, the weight comes right back. It takes time to burn fat and lose weight, there's no doubt about this. It's evident that this kind of weight loss is most likely to be that of fluid and not fat. The moment people go back to their former lifestyle and eating habit, the weight will be back in a matter of time, except if this is long term diet.

In essence, if you are not the type that skips food on a regular basis, especially during the day, you are very much likely to experience some difficulties such as dizziness, headaches, nausea, inability to concentrate

CHAPTER SEVEN

HOW TO FOLLOW SIRTFOODDIET STEP BY STEP

It is simple. The diet comprises two phases for a total period of three weeks. When this is complete, you can then begin to **sirtfy** your diet by combining as many of the Sirtfoods of your choice as you like in your daily meals. There are about top 20 Sirtfoods including the addition of other foods and ingredients. Majority of these foods and ingredients are quite easy to come by.

Phases Involved in SIRTFOOD DIET

The diet is in two phases. Namely:

- First phase, and
- Second phase.

First Phase

The first phase also known as the initial stage. This is for a period of seven days. During this phase, calorie intake is limited to 1,000kcal on a daily basis for a period of three days. Three green juices which include kale, lemon, rocket, celery, green tea and parsley and; and a SIRTFOOD which include chicken and kale curry, prawn stir fry with buckwheat noodles, turkey escalope with parsley, sage and capers. These are the only acceptable meals you can consume.

Beginning from day four till day seven, the calorie intake is increased to 1500kcal, comprising of two green juices and two SIRTFOOD meals daily. Health wise, the diet contains healthy meals and good for the health. It only downside is the restricted calorie and limited choice of food and the guidelines must be filed judiciously in order to achieve the desired result.

Second Phase

For the second phase, this is called the maintenance stage. It is for a period of two weeks (14 days). And this is where the magic lies. Although, this stage is not really focusing on losing weight per se, it's about enjoying the foods nature has provided for us. For this phase, three SIRTFOOD meal is recommended along with two SIRTFOOD snacks and one green juice.

CHAPTER EIGHT

HOW TO COMBINE FOOD FOR OPTIMAL NUTRITION – HOW TO BUILD YOUR OWN RECIPE

When you are particular about the kind of food you eat and the nutritional value they have, the most important thing to consider is not just what passes through your mouth to your stomach, but how your body is able to absorb those nutrients and make better use of them.

The addition of colored and nice looking fruits and vegetables will no doubt give us more nutrients in our meals. But we shouldn't forget the absorption of these nutrients. The body's ability to absorb nutrients from diet known as bioavailability is important just as the nutrients content contained in the food we eat.

There are foods that when combined together with other foods, research indicates can assist your body in absorbing their nutrients efficiently. The believe is that when two specific foods or dm drinks are combined together, they have more beneficial effects on your body than if any of them is consumed alone. This is what is termed **food synergy.** Food synergy explains why we humans develop a taste for consuming some things together and the interaction that exists between them in benefiting our body system and general health. In essence, the best possible way to improve bioavailability of nutrients in our meals is to always remember nutrients synergy relationship when deciding on menus.

When the pairing of two different ingredients improves the body's overall health and its functions, nutrient synergies are said to have taken place.

Below are the combination of some foods that can help your body to optimize their nutritional value. You can as well build your own recipe from this food combo.

I. **Quinoa and Red Pepper**

Quinoa is very rich in fibre, iron and protein. The only deficiency in this type of iron is that it's not easily absorbed by the body. This is not for quinoa alone but for other plant-based foods. The iron present in plant based foods called non-heme iron is not very easy to absorb as compared to the heme-iron present in meat based foods.

Thus, the combination of quinoa and red pepper which has a high percentage of vitamin C will enhance the absorption of iron to a greater extent. This means that when a food rich in vitamin C is combined with any food containing non-heme iron, the iron will be converted into a form that will be easily absorbed. Other combination in this category are lentils and sweet potato, leafy greens and lemon juice, tempeh and broccoli.

Iron absorption is usually blocked by tannins. Tannins are a plant compound present in coffee, peppermint tea, cranberries, red wine, cocoa etc. Although, tannins have certain health benefits but they are known to always decrease the absorption of non-heme iron. It's recommended not to consume any of the foods that contains tannins when eating.

II. **Fresh Cooked Tomatoes and Avocados**

Pairing healthy fats like those found in olive oil with some vegetables can assist your body in absorbing antioxidants. This is also true with the combination of cooked tomatoes with avocados. This is a good source of healthy fat and antioxidants.

III. **Olive Oil and Roasted Sweet Potatoes**

Sweet potato is a good source of Vitamin A olive oil is a good source of healthy fat. Fat soluble vitamins which include vitamins A, D,E and K are easily absorbed when combined with healthy fat. Healthy fat like olive oil, walnut oil, avocado , including nuts and seeds enhances the body's ability to store and absorb fat-soluble vitamins. Another good combination includes kale salad topped with avocado dressing.

IV. **Black Pepper and Turmeric**

Black pepper is effective in the potency and absorption of curcumin. Curcumin is a major anti-inflammatory compound found in turmeric. Curcumin can help in the prevention and treatment of inflammation such as arthritis, Alzheimer's etc. Other combinations in this category include Indian spices, cauliflower and potatoes, baked salmon and cayenne spice etc.

V. **Roast Chicken with Roasted Brussels Sprout**

Both sulforaphanes and selenium perform efficiently when paired together. Sulforaphanes and selenium are good antioxidants and the combination of these duo will increase their antioxidants power. Selenium can be found in food like mushrooms, poultry and so on.

VI. **Salmon and Kale**

The body needs a high amount of vitamin D so it can easily absorb calcium. Calcium is needed for building strong bones and muscles. Salmon is rich in vitamin D while kale is rich in calcium. These two make a perfect food combination. Other sources of vitamin D and calcium combination are tuna and broccoli, egg and cheese. Supplementing calcium is found to have some risks. Therefore, calcium derived directly from food is more preferable.

VII. **Tofu and Dandelion Greens**

Tofu is a rich source of calcium while dandelion greens is a source of inulin. Inulin is a kind of fibre that's responsible for stimulating the levels of the good bacteria in the digestive system. It also helps the bones to absorb calcium easily. When you stir fry both tofu and dandelion greens, you get to supply your body with enough calcium and inulin.

VIII. **Broccoli and Mustard**

Raw broccoli is rich in sulforaphane that has abundant of cancer-fighting properties. But if cooked, the enzyme producing sulforaphane called myrosinase is destroyed. The best way to go about this is to pair both broccoli and mustard together or with another raw cruciferous vegetable. The myrosinase present in mustard will suffice for the ones lost in cooked broccoli. Myrosinase enables the body to easily absorb sulforaphane.

IX. **Lemon and Green Tea**

This is a very nice combination. Green tea has abundant antioxidants, which help in regulating metabolism rate and prevent dehydration. When green tea is combined with lemon, it enables the body to absorb increased amount of antioxidants than when green tea is taken alone.

Other food combinations include: tomato and soy, citrus and iron, vegetables and healthy fat, baked salmon and turmeric, strawberries combine with oatmeal, blueberries with strawberries,

In a nutshell, pairing some particular foods will supply your body with more of some nutrients. This is quite vital most especially if you are suffering from a major deficiency. There are a lot of food combinations that don't work that some brands are promoting. Provided that you know your onions, you should be able to identify what works best for you and what doesn't.

CHAPTER NINE

QUESTIONS AND ANSWERS

Am I Supposed To Exercise During Phase 1?

Engaging in physical exercise is among the things you can do to support your wellbeing and doing so will also help in your weight loss goal in the diet Phase 1. Regular exercise is encouraged during this phase but don't overdo it. Maintain your normal comfort zone. Doing intense exercise may put more stress on your body. But exercise is not a must in this phase. Allow the diet to do the work and just focus on following diet guidelines

I Have A Slim Body Shape, Am I Good To Follow The Diet?

Anyone that's already underweight is not supposed to follow the Phase 1 of this diet. Know your actual weight to know whether or not you are underweight. You will need to calculate your BMI. If you already know your height and weight, this will be easier to calculate. Anyone with a BMI of 18.5 is not recommended to follow the Phase of this diet. If your BMI is within the range 18.5 to 20, caution is needed if you want to follow this diet. The diet alone can decrease your BMI. Also note that being underweight can affect your overall health and this can be at the risk of some health problems. Hence, if you are already underweight, this diet is not recommended for you.

Am I Going To Feel Weak During The Phase 1 Of This Diet?

The Sirtfood diet's two phases consist of highly nutritious foods that have just the right number of compounds that most people are not even used to getting in their everyday meals. When going through this kind of nutritional change, some kind of reaction is expected in some people. The kind of reaction you can have may include dizziness, slight headache, tiredness. But if any of these symptoms persists and becomes chronic, you are advised to see a physician. There's never be a complaint as regards a chronic reaction about this diet. And even those that experience mild symptoms feel much better within a matter of days with a renewed strength and vitality.

Is Supplement Allowed During When Following This Diet?

Using dietary supplements while observing this diet is not recommended except it's recommended by a doctor. And this is mainly because the Sirtfoods already have numerous natural botanical compounds in them so supplementing for any kind of nutrient is not needed. In fact, supplementing for nutritional nutrients when undergoing this diet can actually hinder the effectiveness of the diet and can also cause a reaction. It's better to get any of the nutrients you are lacking in a balanced diet instead of supplementing them.

Can I Repeat The Two Phases On A Regular Basis?

If you wish to repeat the two phases at intervals, it's allowed. This shows you are consistent with the diet. However, most people often realise that they don't need to repeat the Phase 1 of the diet at a close interval. Repeating it at every three months interval is a good one. While for the Phase 2, you can repeat it as many times as you wish since this in itself is an eating habit. With SIRTFOOD Diet, you are not supposed to see yourself as being on a diet. It's a changing period whereby you switch from an old way or habit to a new and positive one.

I've Achieved My Target Weight, Do I Still Continue With The Diet?

This is saying a big congratulations to you. Thumbs up to you. Anyways, since you have reached your target weight, there should be no restriction on your calorie intake anymore and the diet is no longer binding on you. But we still recommend that you continue eating enough SIRTFOOD so as to continue supplying your body with the right amount of nutrients. Don't swerve from this habit as it can make all your effort go in vain. So therefore, continue feeding your body with super rich Sirtfoods and you will thank yourself for it.

What Does The Term Superfoods Means And Can I Include Them In Diet?

There's nothing spectacular about the term superfoods. Neither is it a scientific term, it's just a slogan developed to market the SIRTFOOD Diet. All the Sirtfoods are superfoods. So if you are already following the diet then, you are already eating the superfoods.

Can Children Observe This Diet Too?

This is not a diet designed for children, but the Phase 2 of the diet was defined with family in mind. Majority of the Sirtfoods are low in salt; children need an adequate amount of salt to enhance their growth. Nonetheless, many of the foods are good for children except the green juice. It's highly concentrated for fat burning and this is not ideal for children. Coffee is not also recommended for them and be careful with the amount of pepper you include in the meals.

I've Completed The Phase 2, Do I Still Keep Drinking The Morning Green Juice?

Long term consumption is what we recommend for the green juice. It's a fantastic juice that allows you start our day vibrant and energetic. So, we recommend you continue drinking the green juice. Also, you can switch to any of the SIRTFOOD juice as well.

I'm On Medications, Can I Follow The Diet?

As mentioned earlier, Sirtfood diet is good for almost everyone. However, it has a powerful effect, which can interact with the processes underlined in some health issues and medications. Ideally, some medications don't go well with the Phase 1 of the diet because of the fasting procedure. It's not also advisable that you stop your medication for the time being just so you can follow this diet. Therefore, talk to your medical practitioner for advice.

I'm Overweight, Is The Sirtfood DietFor Me?

Exactly! This diet is for you. But not really for everyone. Being overweight and obese is linked with high risk of many health conditions. But with SIRTFOOD Diet, this can be managed. The diet will help to protect you against chronic health issues associated with being overweight and obese.

CHAPTER TEN

A 7- DAY MEAL PLAN

This is a simple 7-day meal plan for a perfect SIRTFOOD Diet, with 3 recipes per day: one meal plan for breakfast, one meal plan for lunch and one meal plan for dinner which makes it a total of 21. In addition, also included is the daily snack meal plan.

- **Day one**

Breakfast : Soy yogurt with mixed berries, chopped walnut and dark chocolate

Lunch. : A SIRTFOOD salad made with kale, celery, apple, parsley, walnut topped with olive oil mixed with lemon juice and ginger

Dinner : Stir fry prawns with kale and buckwheat noodles

Snack : Celery and hummus

Additional: A SIRTFOOD green juice

- **Day two**

Breakfast : Kale omelette

Lunch : Rocket salad with tuna, tomatoes and cucumber dressed in olive oil

Dinner : Turmeric baked salmon

Snack : Walnut

Additional: A SIRTFOOD green juice

- **Day three**

Breakfast: Fruit smoothie made with rolled oats and soy milk

Lunch : Grilled fish with buckwheat salad

Dinner : Chicken and buckwheat noodles stir fry

Snack : Coffee

Additional: A SIRTFOOD green juice

- **Day four**

Breakfast : Muesli with yogurt and blueberries

Lunch : Kale salad with edamame beans and red onions dressed in olive oil

Dinner : Tofu burger with whole grain bread and salad

Snack : Walnut

Additional: A SIRTFOOD green juice

- **Day five**

Breakfast : Kale omelette

Lunch : Spicy chicken curry with whole grain brown rice

Dinner : Veggies packed spicy tofu stir fry with bird's eye chilli

Snack : Dark chocolate

Additional: A SIRTFOOD green juice

- **Day six**

Breakfast : Braised put lentils

Lunch : Coronation chicken salad

Dinner : Date and walnut porridge

Snack : Strawberries and oranges

Additional: A SIRTFOOD green juice

- **Day seven**

Breakfast : Bunless beef burgers with all the trimmings

Lunch : Smoked salmon omelette

Dinner : Prawn arrabiata

Snack : Celery and hummus

Additional: A SIRTFOOD green juice

CHAPTER ELEVEN

TOP 21 RECIPES

Kickstart your way to a positive lifestyle with this sirtfood diet recipe. The recipes are intended to serve as an example for you so you can be able to create your own recipe. This is not a cookbook. The main purpose of this book is to make you understand how the SIRT Diet works and it intends to make you have the top 21 SIRT diet recipe at your disposal to serve as an inspiration in creating your own dishes. These recipes are packed with flavors and foods rich in nutrients that will change the way you eat. Below are the top 21 SIRT recipes.

Baked Salad with Creamy Mint Dressing

Cooking Time: 20 minutes

Serves: 1

Ingredients

Baked Salmon Salad

4 oz salmon fillet

2 oz mixed salad leaves

2 spring onions (finely sliced)

2 radishes (finely sliced)

1 handful of chopped parsley

1 large cucumber (dice into chunks)

Mint Dressing

2 finely chopped mint leaves

1 tsp pure yogurt

Fresh blended black pepper

1 tsp rice vinegar

1 tsp mayonnaise (low-fat)

Salt to taste

Instructions

1. Preheat oven to 180 C.

2. Put the salmon fillet on a baking pan and bake for 15 minutes.

3. While the salmon is in the oven, get a small bowl and pour in the mayonnaise, yogurt, rice vinegar, pepper, mint leave, salt and mix together. Set aside for few minutes until you start to perceive the flavors.

4. On a serving dish, arrange nicely the salmon leaves and spinach, top with parsley, radishes and red onions.

5. Toss the cooked salmon on the salad and top with the dressing.

Buckwheat Noodles with Chicken, Kale and Miso Dressing

Cooking Time:30 minutes

Serves: 3

Ingredients

Noodles

2 handfuls of neatly cut kale leaves

1 tsp coconut oil

5 oz whole buckwheat noodles

1 brown onion (diced)

1 long and thick chilli (finely sliced)

2 tbsp Tamari sauce, must be gluten free.

3 sliced shiitake mushroom

1 medium size chicken breast (sliced/diced)

2 large garlic cloves (diced)

A few pinch of sea salt to taste

Miso Dressing

1 tbsp Tamari sauce

1 tbsp lemon juice or lime juice

11/2 tbsp fresh organic miso

1 tbsp extra virgin olive oil

1 tsp sesame oil

Instructions

1. Boil a medium size water in a saucepan. Pour in the kale and allow to boil for a minute, until it's a bit droopy. Remove from the water and keep aside.

2. Cook the noodles in the hot water as directed on the package. Afterwards, remove and rinse with cold water and put away.

3. Heat 1 tsp coconut oil in a fry pan and add in the shiitake mushroom. Allow to brown and add little sea salt and put aside.

4. Add more coconut oil to the frying pan over a slightly high heat. Add the onions and chilli pepper and allow to sauté for 2 minutes, 3 minutes max.

5. Add the chicken afterwards into the frying pan and allow to cook for 5 minutes, with a continuous stir. Pour in the garlic and the Tamari sauce and add a little water. Leave to cook for 2 minutes and keep striving until the chicken is tenderly cooked.

6. Add the kale and buckwheat noodles and stir together.

7. Mix the miso dressing and spread on the noodles when you are about ending the cooking.

Asian King Prawn Stir Fry with Buckwheat Noodles

Cooking Time: 15 minutes

Serves:1

Ingredients

5 oz shelled prawn, raw king to be precise.

2.5 oz buckwheat noodles

2 tsp Tamari sauce (gluten free)

2 birds eye chilli

100ml chicken stock

3 tsp extra virgin olive oil

1 garlic clove (chopped)

1 tsp ginger (chopped)

1.5 oz kale (chopped)

2.5 oz green beans

1 red onion (sliced)

1 celery leaf

2 celery leaves (sliced)

Instructions

1. Cooking noodles in a boiling water as instructed on the package. When it's tenderly cooked, drain and keep aside.

2. Bring a frying pan to heat over a medium heat, add the prawns, 1 teaspoon each of the tamari sauce and extra virgin olive oil and allow to cook for 3 minutes. Remove the prawns from the pan and set aside. Clean the pan with a kitchen wipe.

3. Add the remaining oil to the frying pan and pour in the garlic, ginger, red onion, chilli pepper, kale, green beans, celery and allow to fry over a medium heat for about 3 minutes.

4. Pour in the stock and allow the vegetable to cook thoroughly and taste crunchy.

5. Add the noodles, prawns, celery leaves to the mixed vegetables and allow to simmer for few minutes.

6. Remove from the heat and serve hot.

Coronation Chicken Salad

Cooking Time: 5 minutes

Serves: 1

Ingredients

4 oz cooked breast chicken, cut into small pieces

1 tsp blended turmeric

2.5 oz pure yogurt

1 bird's eye chilli

1 tsp chopped coriander

¼ lemon juice

6 ½ walnuts (chopped)

½ tsp curry

1 oz rocket (for serving)

2 medium size red onions (diced)

1 medjool date (neatly chopped)

Instructions

1. Mix together the yogurt, spices, coriander, lemon juice in a clean bowl and mix gently.
2. Add all the other ingredients and mix together.
3. Serve with rocket.

SIRTFOOD Mushroom Scramble Eggs

Cooking Time: 10 minutes

Serves: 1

Ingredients

1 oz kale (chopped)

A large handful of parsley (chopped)

2 eggs

1 tsp curry

A handful of sliced button mushroom

1 tsp extra virgin olive oil

1 tsp turmeric

½ birds eye chilli

Instructions

1. Mix together in a bowl the curry pans turmeric powder. Add a little water and mix till you get a fine and smooth paste.

2. Bring kale to a steam for about 3 minutes.

3. Pour the olive oil in a frying pan and allow to heat then pour in the bird's eye chilli and mushroom and leave to fry for 2 minutes. Allow to turn brown then add the eggs, above paste and leave to simmer. Add the kale and leave to cook for few more minutes.

Sesame Chicken Salad

Cooking Time: 10 minutes

Serves: 2

Ingredients

3 oz baby kale (chopped)

A large handful of parsley (chopped)

1 tbsp sesame seed

½ red onions (sliced)

5 oz of chicken (cooked and shredded)

1 cucumber, peeled, with no seed and sliced.

2 oz pak choi

Dressing

1 tsp sesame oil

1 tsp honey

1 tsp extra virgin olive oil

2 tsp soy sauce

1 lime (juiced)

Instructions

1. Pour the sesame seed in a frying pan and allow to fry for like 2 minutes thereabout. Remove from frying pan when it's slightly brown and set aside.

2. Mix together the remaining sesame oil, olive oil, honey, lime juice and soy sauce in a bowl and set aside. This is the Dressing.

3. Pour the pak choi, cucumber, parsley, kale and red onion in another mixing bowl and mix together. Add the dressing mixture together with this and mix together, until it's well combined.

4. Pour the sesame seed. Serve and add the shredded chicken.

Smoked Salmon Omelette

Cooking Time: 10 minutes

Serves: 1

Ingredients

3.5 oz smoked salmon (sliced)

0.35 oz chopped rocket

1 tsp extra virgin olive oil

2 medium size eggs

½ capers

1 tsp parsley.

Instructions

1. Break the eggs in a bowl and whisk gently.

2. Pour into the egg capers, parsley, salmon, rocket and mix well.

3. Heat the olive oil in a frying pan and allow it to get very hot. Then, pour the egg in the hot oil and spread evenly with a spatula

4. Reduce the heat to low and leave to cook.

5. Use the spatula to smooth the edges and fold the omelette into two then serve.

Salmon SIRT Salad

Cooking Time: 5 minutes

Serves: 2

Ingredients

1.6 oz rocket

0.35 oz chopped parsley

0.35 oz chopped celery leaves

1 large tbsp medjool date

0.7 oz sliced red onion

0.5 oz chopped walnuts

¼ lemon juice

1 tsp capers

1 tsp extra virgin olive oil

2.8 oz chopped avocado

3.5 oz smoked salmon

0.7 oz sliced celery

Instructions

1. Arrange all the Salad leaves in a large serving plate .
2. Add the other ingredients in mixing bowl and mix together gently.
3. Serve the mixture on the leaves.

SIRT Muesli

Cooking Time: 5 minutes

Serves: 2

Ingredients

0.7 oz buckwheat flakes

3.5 oz Plain Greek yogurt

0.7 oz medjool date (finely chopped)

0.35 oz cocoa nibs

3.5 oz chopped strawberries

0.5 oz Coconut flakes

9.35 buckwheat puffs

Direction

In a large mixing bowl, pour in all the ingredients, leaving out the yogurt and strawberries until when you are ready to serve it.

SIRT Fruit Salad

Cooking Time: 10 minutes

Serves: 1

Ingredients

Half cup of fresh green tea

10 blueberries

1 orange

10 red grapes, seedless

1 Apple, chopped and cored

1 tsp honey

Method

1. Add the honey into the green tea and stir. Add the orange juice from half of the orange and keep inside the fridge to cool.

2. Chop the remaining orange in a clean bowl, add all the remaining ingredients and mix together.

3. Bring out the green tea from the fridge and put the mixture on it. Set aside to steep for a while.

4. Serve when properly steeped.

Kale and Black Currant Smoothie

Cooking Time: 5 minutes

Serves: 1

Ingredients

A cup of warm green tea

1 ripe banana

2 tsp honey

6 ice cubes

10 baby kale leaves, without stalk

1.4 oz blackcurrant

Direction

1. Add honey to the green tea and stir.
2. Add all the ingredients together in a food processor and blend.
3. Serve cold.

Green Tea Smoothie

Cooking Time: 5 minutes

Serves: 1

Ingredients

2 tsp matcha green tea powder

A pack of milk

2 tsp honey

2 ripe bananas

6 ice cubes

½ vanilla bean paste

Direction

Blend all the ingredients together in a food processor and serve.

Turmeric Baked Salmon

Cooking Time: 20 minutes

Serves: 2

Ingredients

5 oz skinned salmon

¼ lemon juice

1 tsp turmeric

1 tsp extra virgin olive oil

Spicy Sauce

0.5 oz celery

1 garlic clove

1 large chopped red onion

1 tsp curry powder

1 large tomato, diced into 8 pieces

1 tsp extra virgin olive oil

1 tsp parsley, finely chopped

A medium size canned green beans

1 bird's eye chilli

100ml Chicken stock

Small chopped fresh ginger

Instructions

1. Heat oven at 180 C.

2. As olive oil to a frying pan and allow to heat on a low heat. Add the onions, celery, garlic, chilli, ginger and fry for 2 minutes. Mix in the curry powder and allow to fry for a few seconds.

3. Pour in the tomatoes, green beans and chicken stock and leave to simmer for few more minutes.

4. Mix together the lemon juice, olive oil and turmeric and apply the mixture on the salmon. Arrange on a baking tray and bake for 10 minutes.

5. Sprinkle the parsley spicy sauce and serve with the salmon.

Buckwheat Pasta Salad

Cooking Time: 5 minutes

Serves: 1

Ingredients

1.75 oz buckwheat pasta

A handful of rocket

Half sliced avocado

0.7 oz pine nuts

10 olives

8 cherry tomatoes

1 tsp extra virgin olive oil

Small handful basil leaves

Instructions

Mix all the ingredients together in a bowl, leaving out the pine nuts. When thoroughly mixed, sprinkle the pine nuts on top. Then serve.

Greek Salad Skewers

Cooking Time: 5

Serves: 1

Ingredients

2   wooden skewers

1   yellow pepper, diced

2   3.5oz feta, diced into 8 pieces

8 medium size cherry tomatoes

3.5 oz cucumber, cut into four pieces

½ red onions, cut into 8 pieces

8 large size black olives

Dressing

½ lemon juice

½ garlic clove, mashed

Oregon leaves

1 tsp extra virgin olive oil

Basil leaves

A few pinch black pepper

Salt to taste.

Method

1. Soak the skewers in water for 30 minutes before you begin cooking.

2. Mix the skewers with all the salad ingredients and mix properly.

3. Add all the dressing ingredients in another bowl and mix too.

4. When properly mixed, pour over the skewers and serve.

Grape and Melon Juice

Cooking Time: 5 minutes

Serves: 1

Ingredients

½ finely chopped seedless cucumber

3.5 oz cantaloupe melon (cut into big size)

3.5 red grapes (seedless)

Few spinach leaves

Direction

1. Combine all the ingredients together in a juicer and blend until smooth.

2. Serve cold.

Prawn Arrabbiata

Cooking Time: 15 minutes

Serves: 2

Ingredients

5 oz buckwheat noodles

5 oz cooked king prawns

1 tsp extra virgin olive oil

Arrabbiata Sauce

0.5 oz chopped celery

A can of chopped tomatoes

1   birds eye chilli

2   tbsp white wine

1 garlic clove

1 large red onions, chopped

1 tbsp parsley, chopped

1 tbsp dried mixed herbs

1 tsp extra virgin olive oil

Instructions

1. Boil pasta in a pot as directed on the package.
2. While the pasta is cooking, get a frying pan, add olive oil and allow to heat on a low heat. Add the garlic, chilli, onion, dried herbs and celery and allow to fry for about 2 minutes.

3. Increase the heat and pour in the white wine. This is optional. Cook for 2 minutes.

4. Add the tomatoes and allow to simmer for 15 minutes. Add a little water if required.

5. Check the pasta, drain the water if properly cooked and add olive oil to it then set aside.

6. Add the cooked prawns to the sauce with the parsley and allow to cook for few minutes.

7. Add the pasta and sauce together.

8. Serve hot.

Fragrant Asian Hotspot

Cooking Time: 15 minutes

Serves: 2

Ingredients

1.4 oz sushi ginger

500ml Chicken stock

3.5 oz raw tiger prawns

3.5 oz tofu

1.75   oz bean sprout

1.75 oz broccoli

½ carrot, neatly cut into matchstick size

½ lime juice

1 crushed star anise

1 tbsp miso paste

Small handful coriander and stalks

Small handful parsley and stalks

1.75   oz water chestnuts

1.75 oz rice noodles

I tsp tomato purée

Direction

1. In a large sauté pan, add the coriander stalks, star anise, lime juice, parsley stalks, chicken stock, tomato purée and cook for 8 minutes.

2. Pour in the tofu, broccoli, water chestnut, prawns, noodles, carrot and cook until tender.

3. When the mixture is tenderly cooked, turn off the heat and add the sushi ginger and miso paste.

4. Sprinkle with parsley and coriander leaves before serving.

Kale Edamame and Tofu Curry

Cooking Time: 15 minutes

Serves: 2

Ingredients

1 large chopped onion

½ powdered turmeric

½ powdered cumin

½ tsp cayenne pepper

1 red chilli

4 grated garlic cloves

1 tsp paprika

8.75 oz dried red lentils

8.75 kale leaves

1.75 oz soya edamame beans

7 oz diced tofu

1 tsp rapeseed oil

A litre of boiled water

1 tsp salt

2 chopped tomatoes

1 lime juice

1 large grated ginger

Method

1. Pour oil in a deep pan over a low heat and add onions. Allow the onion to cook for roughly 5 minutes then add the chilli pepper, garlic and ginger and leave for two minutes to cook.

2. Toss in the cayenne, cumin, turmeric, paprika and salt. Mix very well and add the red beans and stir.

3. Add boiling water and leave to cook until it's getting thicker, more like porridge.

4. Pour in the tomatoes, soya beans and tofu and simmer for few minutes.

5. Add the kale leaves and lime juice and leave to simmer again.

6. Serve when ready.

Choc Chip Granola

Cooking Time: 40 minutes

Serves: 3

Ingredients

7   oz jumbo oats

1.75 oz pecans

2   tbsp olive oil

1 tbsp dark sugar

2 tbsp rice malt syrup

1.4 oz butter

2.1 oz dark chocolate

Instructions

1. Heat oven at 140 C.
2. Wrap a large baking tray with a parchment.
3. Add the oats and pecans in a bowl and mix together.
4. In a small pan, heat the olive oil, brown sugar, malt syrup, butter until all of them have melted. Remove from the heat so the content won't get boil. Boiling the content is not the idea.
5. Now, pour the syrup on top of the oats and spread evenly.
6. Spread out the granola on the baking tray, ensuring there's space between the mixture.
7. Allow to bake for 20 minutes until it has turned golden. Then set aside to cool.

8. When it's cool, divide any lumps that's too big and then mix the content with the chocolate chips.

9. Pour the granola into a tight container to prevent air from passing through.

10. Keep it for a period of two weeks before eating it.

SIRTFOOD Miso Marinated Cod with Stir Fry Greens and Sesame

Cooking Time: 30 minutes

Serves: 2

Ingredients

7 cod fillet, skinless

2 tbsp mirin

0.7 oz red onion

0.7 oz miso

1.05 oz buckwheat

1 chopped bird's eye chilli

1 tbsp extra virgin olive oil

2 1 tsp chopped ginger

Small handful parsley

1.75 kale

1 garlic clove

2.1 oz green beans

1 tsp tamari

1 tsp powdered turmeric

1 tsp sesame seed

Instructions

1. Add miso, 1 tsp olive oil and moron together and spread on the cod. Then leave to marinate afterwards.

2. Heat oven at 220 C.

3. Put the cod in the oven to bake for few minutes.

4. In another pan, pour the buckwheat and cook as directed on the packet. Add turmeric after a little while.

5. Add the remaining oil in a large frying pan. Add the onions and fry for a while. Pour in the garlic, ginger, celery, kale, green beans and chilli. Fry until the kale is properly cooked. If needed, you may need to add a little water to make it cook properly.

6. When the buckwheat is ready, drain and set aside.

7. Add the tamari, sesame seed and parsley to the stir fry.

8. Top the buckwheat with the stir fry and serve with the cod and greens.

These recipes are intended to serve as an example so you can be able to easily create your own recipe. All the above mentioned Sirtfoods are rich in nutrients that your body craves for.

CONCLUSION

The Sirtfood diet centres on research conducted on SIRTUINS, a family of protein that stimulates many functions in the body. These are foods that when consumed, they can help activate this protein in our body to produce additional amount of the protein. This diet may be effective in losing weight because it's strictly based on calorie restriction. It advocates eating low calories during a three week period of following the diet. The diet is simple to follow as it contains just two phases with detailed instructions.

The SIRTUINS protein is said to be play significant role in reducing inflammation, preventing the growth of tumors and reducing the risk of heart disease and other cardiovascular related disease.

Weight gain is associated with different health related issues including obesity and diabetes. This is why it's important that you pay adequate attention to your body weight. Weight loss and fat burning is not something that can achieve over night but with dedication and consistency, it's possible to achieve weight loss over a period of time. While it's good to engage in physical activities, caution must be taken. Too much of high intense exercise can put stress on the body which is not what you really what for yourself.

Finally, don't forget that dieting and exercise go hand in hand in any weight loss program. When you eat the right kind of food and you engage in activities that support weight loss, you will definitely achieve your target weight.

Finally, we hope you find the top 21 Sirtfood diet recipe will be useful in developing your own recipe. Also, feel free to combine any of the food combinations mentioned to get optimal nutritional value that will benefit your health.

Reference

Riveros-McKay et al. 2019. "Genetic Architecture of human thinness compared to severe obesity. PLOS Genetics".

Salas-Salvado J et al. 2014. The Prevention of diabetes with Mediterranean diets.

Radak et al.2013."Redox-regulating sirtuins in aging, caloric restriction and exercise".

Haigis MC and Guarente LP. 2006. "Mammaliansirtuins-emerging roles in physiology, aging and calorie restriction".

Ibarrola-Jurado N et al. 2013. "Cross sectional assessment of nut consumption and obesity, metabolic syndrome and other cardio metabolic risk factors".

EStruch R et al. 2013. "Primary prevention of cardiovascular disease with a Mediterranean diet".

https://www.healthline.com/nutrition/Sirtfood-diet#section6

https://www.getthegloss.com/article/what-a-dietician-really-thinks-of-the-the-sirt-food-diet

https://www.healthyfood.com/advice/the-Sirtfood-diet/

https://greatist.com/health/how-to-lose-body-fat#tl-dr

https://www.google.com/search?q=the+importance+of+exercise&rlz=1CDGOYI_enNG822NG822&oq=the+importance+of+exercise+&aqs=chrome..69i57j0l3.9954j0j4&hl=en-US&sourceid=chrome-mobile&ie=UTF-8

CPSIA information can be obtained
at www.ICGtesting.com
Printed in the USA
LVHW101531101120
671304LV00010B/336